NATURAL WAYS TO TREAT ERECTILE DYSFUNCTION

Dr. Bayo

Copyright © 2019 by **Dr.Bayo**

All rightsreserved. Printed in the United States of America. No part of this book maybeused or reproduced in anymannerwhatsoeverwithoutwritten permission except in the case of briefquotationsem- bodied in critical articles or reviews.

TABLE OF CONTENTS

NATURAL WAYS TO TREAT ERECTILE DYSFUNCTION I

INTRODUCTION 5

CHAPTER ONE 8

   WHAT IS ERECTILE DYSFUNCTION? 8
      What are are symptoms of erectile dysfunction? 8
      Causes of erectile dysfunction 9

CHAPTER TWO 12

   HOW TO DIAGONISED ERECTILE DYSFUNCTION 12
      Nocturnal penile tumescence (NPT) test 12
      Treatments for Erectile Dysfunction 13
   ORAL DRUGS (PDE5 INHIBITORS) 14
   TESTOSTERONE THERAPY 15
   VACUUM ERECTION DEVICE 15
   INTRACAVERNOSAL (ICI) AND URETHRA (IU) THERAPIES 15
   SELF-INJECTION THERAPY 16
   INTRAURETHRAL (IU) THERAPY 17
   SURGICAL TREATMENT 17
      Semi rigid Implant (Bendable) 18
      Inflatable Implant 18
   WHAT IS THE SURGERY LIKE? 18
   CLINICAL TRIALS 20
   SUPPLEMENTS 20
   ALTERNATIVE TREATMENT OF ERECTILE DYSFUNCTION 21
      Prostatic massage 21
      Acupuncture 21
      Pelvic floor muscle exercises 22
      Lifestyle changes and diet 22
   MEDICATION FOR ERECTILE DYSFUNCTION 23

CHAPTER THREE 25

- Risk factors of Erectile Dysfunction... 25

CHAPTER FOUR 27
- How does age affect incidence of Erectile Dysfunction? 27
- Natural ways to overcome Erectile Dysfunction 28
- Frequently asked question on Erectile Dysfunction 30
  - How do I know my ED is physical and not mental?..................................... 30
  - If I worry about being able to get an erection, can I make a bad condition worse?.. 30
  - Can I combine treatment options? 30
  - I was fine until I began taking this new drug, what should I do?............. 30

ABOUT THE AUTHOR 31

ACKNOWLEDGMENTS 32

Introduction

During sexual arousal, nerves allow chemicals that high blood flow into the penis. Blood flows into two erection chambers in the penis, made of spongy muscle tissue (the corpus cavernosum). The corpus cavernosum chambers are not hollow.

During erection, the spongy tissues relax and trap blood. The blood pressure in the chambers makes the penis firm, causing an erection. When a man has an orgasm, a second set of nerve signals reach the penis and cause the muscular tissues in the penis to contract and blood is released back into a man's circulation and the erection comes down.

When you are not sexually aroused, the penis is soft and limp. Men may observe that the size of the penis different from warmth, cold or worry; this is normal and reflects the balance of blood coming into and leaving the penis.

Erectile dysfunction, or ED, is the most common sex issues that men report to their medical personnel. It affects as many as 30 million men.

ED is defined as issues getting or keeping an erection that's firm enough for sex.

Though it's not rare for a man to have some problems with erections from time to time, ED that is progressive or occurs routinely with sex is not normal, and it should be treated.

ED can occur:

- Most often when blood flow in the penis is limited or nerves are harmed
- With stress or emotional reasons
- As an early warning of a more serious illness, like: atherosclerosis (hardening or blocked arteries), heart disease, high blood pressure or high blood sugar from Diabetes

Erectile dysfunction is the inability to get and keep an erection firm or active for sex.

Having erection issue from time to time is not necessarily a cause for worry. If an erectile dysfunction is an ongoing problem, however, it can cause stress, affect your self confidence and add to relationship problems. Problems getting or keeping an erection can also be a sign of an underlying health condition that needs treatment and risk factors for heart disease.

If you are worried about erectile dysfunction, contact your medical personnel, even if you are embarrassed. Sometimes, curing an underlying condition is enough to bring back erectile dysfunction. In most cases, medications or other direct treatments might be needed.

Occasional ED isn't uncommon. Many men experience it during times of stress. Frequent ED can be a symptoms of health problems that need treatment. It can also be a sign of emotional or relationship difficulties that may need to be addressed by a professional.

Not every male sexual issues are caused by ED. Other types of male sexual dysfunction include:

- premature ejaculation
- delayed or absent ejaculation

Chapter One

WHAT IS ERECTILE DYSFUNCTION?

Erectile dysfunction, also known as ED or impotence, is the inability to attain or maintain an erection of the penis adequate for the sexual satisfaction of both partners. It can be devastating and worrysome to the self-esteem of a man and of his partner. As many as 30 million American men are afflicted on a daily basis, and transient episodes affect nearly all adult males. But almost all men who seek for cure find some measure of relief.

What are are symptoms of erectile dysfunction?

You may have erectile dysfunction if you regularly have:

- trouble getting an erection
- difficulty maintaining an erection during sexual activities
- reduced interest in sex

Other sexual disorders related to ED include:

- premature ejaculation

- delayed ejaculation
- anorgasmia, which is the inability to achieve orgasm after ample stimulation

You should talk to your medical personnel if you have any of these symptoms, especially if they've lasted for two or more months. Your medical personnel can decide if your sexual disorder is caused by an underlying condition that requires treatment.

Causes of erectile dysfunction

There are many possible causes for ED, and they can include both emotional and physical disorders. Some major causes are:

- cardiovascular disease
- diabetes
- hypertension
- hyperlipidemia
- damage from cancer or surgery

- injuries
- obesity or being overweight
- increased age
- stress
- anxiety
- relationship problems
- drug use
- alcohol use
- smoking

ED can be caused by only one of these factors or several. That's why it's very vital to work with your medical personnel so that they can rule out or treat any underlying medical conditions.

An erection is the result of high blood flow into your penis. Blood flow is usually stimulated by either sexual thoughts or direct contact with your penis.

When a man becomes sexually excited, muscles in their penis relax. This relaxation allows for high blood flow through the penile arteries. This blood fills two chambers inside the penis called the corpora cavernosa. As the chambers fill with blood, the penis grows hard. Erection stops when the muscles contract and the accumulated blood can flow out through the penile veins.

ED can occur because of issues at any stage of the erection process. For example, the penile arteries may be too destroyed to open properly and allow blood in.

Chapter Two

How to Diagonised Erectile Dysfunction

Your medical personnel will ask you questions about your symptoms and health history. They may conduct tests to decide if your symptoms are caused by an underlying condition. You should expect a physical exam where your medical personnel will listen to your heart and lungs check your blood pressure, and check your testicles and penis. They may also recommend a rectal exam to examine your prostate. In addittion, you may need blood or urine examination to rule out other conditions.

Nocturnal penile tumescence (NPT) test

An NPT test is conducted using a portable, battery-powered device that you wear on your thigh while you're sleeping. The device evaluates the quality of nocturnal erections and stores the data, which your medical personnel can later access. Your medical personnel can use this data to better understand your penis function and ED.

Nocturnal erections are erections that happens while you're sleeping, and they're a normal part of a healthily functioning penis.

Treatments for Erectile Dysfunction

Non-invasive treatments are often tried first. Most of the best-known treatments for ED work well and are safe. Still, it helps to ask your medical personnel about side effects that could result from each option:

- Oral drugs or pills known as phosphodiesterase type-5 inhibitors are most often prescribed in the U.S. for ED (Viagra, Cialis, Levitra, Stendra)
- Testosterone Therapy (when low testosterone is detected in blood testing)
- Penile Injections (ICI, intracavernosal Alprostadil)
- Intraurethral medication (IU, Alprostadil)
- Vacuum Erection Devices
- Penile Implants
- Surgery to bypass penile artery damage for some younger men with a history of severe pelvic trauma. Penile vascular surgery is not recommended for older men with hardened arteries.

Oral Drugs (PDE5 inhibitors)

Drugs known as PDE type-5 inhibitors high the penile blood flow. These are the only oral agents approved in the U.S. by the Food and Drug Administration for the treatment of ED.

- Viagra (sildenafil citrate)
- Levitra (vardenafil HCl)
- Cialis (tadalafil)
- Stendra (avanafil)

For best results, men living with ED use these pills about an hour or two before having sex. The drugs require normal nerve function to the penis. PDE5 inhibitors effect on normal erectile responses helping blood flow into the penis. Use these drugs as directed. About 7 out of 10 men perform well and have better erections. Response rates are reduce for Diabetics and cancer patients.

If you are using nitrates for your heart, you should not take any PDE5 inhibitors. Always speak with your medical personnel before using a PDE5 inhibitor to learn how it might affect your health.

Most times, the side effects of PDE5 inhibitors are mild and often last just a short time. The most common side effects are:

- Headache
- Stuffy nose
- Facial flushing
- Muscle aches

- Indigestion

In few cases, the drug Viagra can cause blue-green shading to vision that lasts for a short time. In few cases, the drug Cialis cans high the back pain or aching muscles in the back. In most cases, the side effects are linked to PDE5 inhibitor effects on other tissues in the body, meaning they are working to high the blood flow to your penis and simultaneously impacting other vascular tissues in your body. These are not 'allergic reactions'.

Testosterone Therapy

In those few cases where a low sex drive and reduce blood levels of Testosterone are at fault for ED, Testosterone Therapy may fix normal erections or assist when combined with ED drugs (PDE type 5 inhibitors).

Vacuum Erection Device

A vacuum erection device is a plastic tube that slips over the penis, making a seal with the skin of the body. A pump at the other end of the tube makes a low-pressure vacuum around the erectile tissue, which results in an erection. An elastic ring is then slipped onto the base of the penis. This holds the blood in the penis (and keeps it hard) for up to 30 minutes. With proper training, 75 out of 100 men can get a working erection using a vacuum erection device.

Intracavernosal (ICI) and Urethra (IU) Therapies

If oral drugs don't work, the drug Alprostadil is approved for use in men with ED. This drug comes in two forms, based on how it is to be used: intracavernosal injection (called "ICI") or through the urethra (called "IU therapy").

Self-Injection Therapy

Alprostadil is injected into the side of penis with a very fine needle. It's of great value to have the first shot in the medical personnel office before doing this on your own. Self-injection lessons should be given in your doctor's office by an experienced professional. The success rate for getting an erection firm enough to have sex is as high as 85% with this treatment. Most men who do not respond to oral PDE5 inhibitors can be 'rescued' with ICI.

ICI Alprostadil may be used as a mixture with two other drugs to treat ED. This additonal therapy called "bimix or trimix" is harder than alprostadil alone and has become standard cure for ED. Only the Alprostadil ingredient is FDA approved for ED. The amount of each drug used can be changed based on the severity of your ED, by an experienced health professional. You will be trained by your medical personnel on how to inject, how much to inject and how to safely raise the drug's dosage if necessary.

ICI therapy often make available a reliable erection, which comes down after 20-30 minutes or with climax. Since the ICI erection is not regulated by your penile nerves, you should not be surprised if the erection lasts after orgasm. The most common side effect of ICI therapy is a prolonged erection. Prolonged erections (>1 hour) can be reversed by a second injection (antidote) in the office.

Men who have penile erections that can last longer than two to four hours should consult an Emergency Room care. Priapism is a prolonged erection, lasting longer than four hours. It is very painful. Failure to undo priapism will lead to permanent penile destruction and uncurable ED.

Intraurethral (IU) Therapy

For IU therapy, a tiny medicated pellet of the drug, Alprostadil, is placed in the urethra (the tube that carries urine out of your body). Using the drug this way means you don't have to give yourself a shot, unfortunately it may not work as well as ICI. Like ICI therapy, IU Alprostadil should be tested in the office, before home usage.

The most common side effects of IU alprostadil are a burning feeling in the penis. If an erection lasts for over four hours, it will require medical attention to make it go down.

Surgical Treatment

The main surgical treatment of ED involves insertion of a penile implant (also called penile prostheses). Because penile vascular surgery is not approved for aging males who have failed oral PDE5 inhibitors, ICI or IU therapies, implants are the next step for these patients. Although placement of a penile implant is a surgery which carries risks, they have the highest rates of success and satisfaction among ED treatment options.

Penile implants are devices that are placed fully inside your body. They make a stiff penis that lets you have normal sex. This is an excellent choice to improve uninterupted intimacy and makes relations more spontaneous.

There are two types of penile implants.

Semi rigid Implant (Bendable)

The easiest kind of implant is produce from two easy-to-bend rods that are most often made of silicone. These silicone rods give the man's penis the firmness needed for sexual penetration. The implant can be bent downward for peeing or upward for sex.

Inflatable Implant

With an inflatable implant , fluid-filled cylinders are placed lengthwise in the penis. Tubing joins these cylinders to a pump placed inside the scrotum (between the testicles). When the pump is engaged, pressure in the cylinders inflate the penis and makes it stiff. Inflatable implants make a normal looking erection and are natural feeling for your partner. Your surgeon may suggest a lubricant for your partner. With the implant, men can control firmness and, sometimes, the size of the erection. Implants free a couple to be spontaneously intimate. There is generally no change to a man's feeling or orgasm.

What is the Surgery Like?

Penile implants are mostly placed under anesthesia. If a patient has a systemic, skin, or urinary tract infection, this surgery should be postponed until all infections are cured. If a man is on blood thinners, then he may need to talk with medical personnel about stopping the medications for elective surgery and healing.

Most often, one small surgical cut is made. The cut is either above the penis where it joins the belly or under the penis where it joins the scrotum. No tissue is removed. Blood loss is typically small. A patient will either go home on the same day or spend one night in the hospital.

Recovery Time after Penile Implants:

- Most men will feel pain and will feel better with a narcotic pain-relief drug for one to two weeks. After the first week, over- the-counter pain drugs (such as acetaminophen or ibuprofen) may be substituted for narcotic pain drugs.
- Discomfort, bruising and swelling after the surgery will last for a few weeks.
- For the first month, men should limit their physical activity. The surgeon will explain when and how much exercises to do during the healing period.

Men most often start having sex with their penile implants

by two months after surgery.

- If there is insisting swelling or pain, the use of the implant may be delayed. The surgeon or medical personnel in the surgeon's office will talk about how toinflate and deflate the implant.
  There are risks to prosthetic surgery and patients are counselled before the procedure. If there is a post-operative infection, the implant will likely be removed. The devices are reliable, but in the case of mechanical malfunction, the device or a part of the device will need to be replaced surgically. If a penile prosthesis is taken away, other non-surgical treatments may no longer work.
  Most men with penile implants and their partners

say that they're satisfied with the results, and they return to more spontaneous intimacy.

Clinical Trials

Most restorative or regenerative cures are under investigation for the future treatment of ED:

- Extracorporeal shock wave therapy (ESWT) - low-intensity shock waves that aim to fix the erectile tissues and help restore natural erections.
- Intracavernosal injection of stem cells - to help cavernous tissue regrowth
- Intracavernosal injection autologous platelet rich plasma (APRP) - to help cavernous tissue regrowth. These are not latest approved by the FDA for ED management, but they may be offered through research studies. Patients who are interested should discuss the risks and benefits of each, as well as costs before starting any clinical trials. Most therapies not endorsed by the FDA are not covered by government or private insurance benefits.

Supplements

Supplements are common and often not expensive than prescription drugs for ED. However, supplements have not been tested to see how well they work or if they are a safe treatment for ED. Patients should know that many over-the-counter drugs have been found on drug testing to have 'bootlegged' PDE 5 Inhibitors as their main ingredient. The amount of Viagra, Cialis, Levitra or

Stendra that may be in these supplements is not under quality control and may differ from pill to pill. The FDA has issued consumer warnings and alerts.

Alternative treatment of Erectile Dysfunction

If your ED is caused by stress, yoga and massage may assist if you find these activities relaxing.

Prostatic massage

Some men use a form of massage therapy called prostatic massage. Practitioners massage the tissues in and around your groin to promote blood flow to your penis. There are limited studies on the efficacy of this type of massage.

Acupuncture

Acupuncture may assistTrusted Source treat psychological ED, though researches are limited and inconclusive. You'll likely need several appointments before you start to notice any improvements. When choosing an acupuncturist, look for a certified practitioner who uses disposable needles and follows U.S. Food and Drug Administration guidelines for needle disposal and sterilization.

Pelvic floor muscle exercises

A small research of 55 men saw improvement to penile function after three months of regular pelvic floor muscles exercises, and after six months, 40 percent of men had regained normal erectile function.

Kegel exercises are a simple exercise you can apply to strengthen your pelvic floor muscles. Here's how you do them:

1. Get to know your pelvic floor muscles. To do this, stop peeing midstream. The muscles you use to do this are your pelvic floor muscles. Your testicles will also rise when you contract these muscles.
2. Now that you know where these muscles are, contract them for 5 to 20 seconds. Then release them.
3. Repeat this exercise 10 to 20 times in a row, three to four times a day.

Lifestyle changes and diet

Healthy lifestyle habits may stop ED, and in some situations bring back the condition:

- Exercise regularly.
- Maintain a low blood pressure.
- Eat a balanced, nutritious diet.
- Maintain a healthy weight.
- Avoid alcohol and cigarettes.
- Reduce your stress.

ED is often related to issues with your blood flow, so maintaining your blood vessel health through exercise and a healthy diet may help lower your risk for ED.

Medication For Erectile Dysfunction

Your medical personnel may prescribe medication to help manage your symptoms of ED. You may need to try diffrent medications before you find a particular one that works. These medications can have side effects. If you're going through unpleasant side effects, talk to your medical personnel. They may be able to approve a different medication.

The following medications stimulate blood flow to your penis to help treat ED:

- alprostadil (Caverject)

- avanafil (Stendra)
- sildenafil (Viagra)
- tadalafil (Cialis)
- testosterone (Androderm)
- vardenafil (Levitra)

Chapter Three

Risk factors of Erectile Dysfunction

As you get older, erections might take longer to grow and might not be as firm. You might need more direct touch to your penis to get and keep an ereection. Various factors can contribute to erectile dysfunction, including;

i. **medical condition**, particularly diabetes or heart condition

Ii. **Tobacco use**, which restricts blood flow to veins arteries, can over time cause chronic health conditions that lead to erectile dysfunction.

Iii. **Being overweight**, especially if you are obese

Iv. **Certain medical treatments**, such as prostrate surgery or radiation treatment for cancer.

V. **Injuries**, particularly if they damage the nerves or arteries that control erections.

Vi.**Medications**, including anti depressants, antihistamines and medication to treat high blood pressure, pain or prostate conditions.

Vii. **Psychological conditions**, such as stress, anxiety or depression.

Viii.**drug and alcohol use**,especially if you are a long term drug user or heavy drinker

Complications

Complications resulting from erectile dysfunction can include;

1.An unsatisfactory sex life
2.Stress or anxiety
3.Embarassment or low self esteem
4. Relationship problems
5.The inability to get your partner pregnant

Chapter Four

How does age affect incidence of Erectile Dysfunction?

Up to 30 million American men are affected by ED, according to the research conducted by National Institute of Diabetes and Digestive and Kidney Diseases. The prevalence of ED increases with age. ED affects:

- 12 percent of men younger than 60
- 22 percent of men in their 60s
- 30 percent of men 70 or older

Although the risk of ED increases with age, ED is not inevitable as you get older. It may be more difficult to get an erection as you age, but that doesn't necessarily mean you will develop ED. In general, the healthier you are, the better your sexual function.

ED can also happen among younger men. A 2013 research found that one in four men seeking their first cure for ED were under the age of 40. The researchers found a stronger correlation between smoking and illicit drug use and ED in men under 40 than among older men. That suggests that lifestyle choices may be a main contributing factor for ED in younger men.

An analysis of studiedTrusted Source on ED in men under 40 found that smoking was a factor for ED among 41 percent of men under the age of 40. Diabetes was the next most common risk factor and was linked to ED in 27 percent of men under 40.

Natural ways to overcome Erectile Dysfunction

Whether you currently suffer from ED or are hoping to sidestep this condition, try these tips to overcome ED for better health and a better sex life.

1. **Start walking.** According to one Harvard study, just 30 minutes of walking a day was linked with a 41% drop in risk for ED. Other study suggests that moderate exercise can assist restore sexual performance in obese middle-aged men with ED.
2. **Eat right.** In the Massachusetts Male Aging Study, eating a diet rich in natural foods like fruit, vegetables, whole grains, and fish ,with fewer red and processed meat and refined grains , lower the likelihood of ED.
3. **Pay attention to your vascular health.** High blood pressure, high blood sugar, high cholesterol, and high triglycerides can all damage arteries in the heart (causing

heart attack), in the brain (causing stroke), and leading to the penis (causing ED). An expanding waistline also contributes. Check with your medical personnel to find out whether your vascular system and thus your heart, brain, and penis is in good shape or needs a tune-up through lifestyle changes and, if necessary, medications.

4. **Size matters, so get slim and stay slim.** A trim waistline is one good defense a man with a 42-inch waist is 50% more likely to have ED than one with a 32-inch waist. Weight reduction can assist fight erectile dysfunction, so getting to a healthy weight and staying there is another good strategy for avoiding or fixing ED. Obesity raises risks for vascular disease and diabetes, two major causes of ED. And excess fat interferes with several hormones that may be part of the issue as well.

5. **Move a muscle, but we're not talking about your biceps.** A strong pelvic floor enhances rigidity during erections and assists keep blood from leaving the penis by pressing on a key vein. In a British trial, three months of twice-daily sets of Kegel exercises (which strengthen these muscles), combined with biofeedback and advice on lifestyle changes quitting smoking, losing weight, limiting alcohol worked far better than just advice on lifestyle changes.

Frequently asked question on Erectile Dysfunction

How do I know my ED is physical and not mental?

It's hard to know. Health providers now realize that most men have an underlying physical cause of ED. For most patients, there are both physical and emotional factors that lead to ED. It is impossible to prove that there is no psychological part to a man's ED.

If I worry about being able to get an erection, can I make a bad condition worse?

Nothing happens in the body without the brain. Worrying about your ability to get an erection can make it difficult to get one. This is called performance anxiety and can be overcome with education and treatment.

Can I combine treatment options?

This is often done. However, only combine treatments after talking with your health care provider about this. Erections can last too long with drug therapy, which is dangerous. Ask your doctor for proper instructions.

I was fine until I began taking this new drug, what should I do?

Never stop or change a prescription medication without first talking with your health care provider.

Many drugs can cause ED, but some cannot be changed because the drug's benefits are too important for you. If you feel sure that a specific drug has caused the ED problem, ask your health care provider if you can change drugs. If you must stay on the drug that is causing the problem, there are ED treatments that can help.

About the Author

Dr. Bayo is a pastor and a medical practioner who studied pharmacy in SefakoMakgatho Health Sciences University (SMU) in South Africa and receive his Phd in Lipscomb University in Missouri-columbia.
He has involved himself into prescriptions and cure of diseases and sickness. He is a solution to many problems amidst its environment such has cancer, stroke infection, erectile dysfuntion, anti-biotic infection, how to reduce your blood pressure and lots more to mention but a little.
He has been eagerly and greatly having impact in the life of msny others in the area of pharmaceutical trainings and has been building people to be pharmaceutically awake in order not to be deceived by fake drug sellers out there.
Other books by Dr. Bayo are: 100% ways to stay healthy

with Moringa and 100% natural ways to treat leukemia.

Acknowledgments

My appreciation goes to God, Almighty for the opportunity to collate this manuscript, and for wisdom he gave me to spread the knowledge around. Also I appreciate everyone that supported me during the compilation, proof reading and publishing of the book

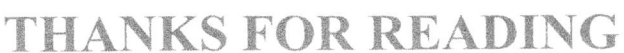

www.ingramcontent.com/pod-product-compliance
Lightning Source LLC
Chambersburg PA
CBHW070909220526
45466CB00005B/2179